My Autologous Stem Cell Transplant

One Patient's Perspective

By Andy Burrows

ISBN: 978-1539701545

Contents

Introduction

I'm publishing this book for all those who have to go through a stem cell transplant as part of their treatment for some serious illness.

My stem cell transplant was an 'autologous peripheral blood stem cell transplant'. I had that at Southampton Hospital in Hampshire, England, at the end of 2015.

'Autologous' means that it involved transplanting my own stem cells, that had been harvested when I was in remission from my cancer.

'Peripheral blood' means that the stem cells were both taken from and injected back into my blood stream. Normally stem cells reside inside the bone marrow, develop into blood cells and come out into the blood stream. However, they can be encouraged to come out to be harvested from the blood stream, and they can flourish if injected back into the blood stream. I guess that's what makes it different to a 'bone marrow transplant', although no one has been able to explain the difference when I ask.

The condition I was being treated for was recurrent follicular non-Hodgkin's lymphoma. I was seriously ill in 2009/10 with high grade Diffuse Large B-Cell lymphoma, and was treated with R-CHOP chemotherapy. I relapsed in 2012 with a low grade form, follicular lymphoma, and then again in 2015. Normally follicular lymphoma is treated as a chronic, but not life threatening, disease, and it can be left untreated for years sometimes. And the fact that it's not normally considered curable is not normally a problem. However, since I was relapsing every couple of years, I was put forward for a stem cell transplant.

The stem cell transplant should give me a chance of being cancer free. We shall see.

The stem cells were harvested after my first relapse, in 2013, when I was confirmed in remission. Since they were not intending to go straight ahead with the transplant, at that time they called it a "rainy day harvest". That "rainy day" came in 2015 with my second relapse.

I posted my cancer journal on my blog[1], over more than six years starting from 2009, covering all three occurrences and culminating with my stem cell transplant. That journal was turned into a book called *Cancer and Me* in 2016. It's what I call the "omnibus edition" of those blog entries.

---

[1] www.andyburrows.me

Being a Christian, I also reflected quite a lot on how I looked at my cancer experience through my faith. And from that came the more autobiographical and reflective book, *Facing Cancer with Faith*. You can find out more about both books at www.andyburrows.me.

I decided to publish this little book as well as the other two, because a stem cell transplant is a big deal in its own right, and those who have to face it normally like to know how other people have coped. The information given to patients beforehand, published by the Lymphoma Association and others, is genuinely great and helpful, but a first-hand account of going through it helps to make it less mysterious and scary. And it gives hope that, even though you know you will feel really rough during the process, people do come out the other side, recover quickly and get back to normal. I used blogs written by other lymphoma sufferers and stem cell transplant patients in a similar way and found them very helpful.

The core chapters included here are unashamedly copied with very little editing from one of my earlier books. There are only so many ways of telling the same story!

So if you're facing an autologous stem cell transplant in the near future I hope that this little book will help you. But however you mentally prepare, I wish you all the best. I hope that your transplant is both successful and free of complications.

Setting the Scene

By way of reminder, an autologous stem cell transplant comes in several stages:

1. Harvest healthy stem cells when you are in remission;
2. High dose chemotherapy to destroy all white blood cells;
3. Infuse stem cells back into blood stream;
4. Recovery and growth of healthy white cells.

As I mentioned in the introduction, my stem cell transplant experience is in two parts. I had a "rainy day" stem cell harvest more than two years before my autologous transplant. Most people, as I understand it, would go straight from harvesting to have the transplant as soon as a bed is available in an appropriate specialist isolation ward. Essentially, though, the overall process is the same.

Since in this book I'm only focusing on the stem cell transplant process, I haven't included any account of my diagnoses, my illnesses or my feelings about them. If you find yourself interested in those parts of my experience, you can read about them in either of my other two books.

However, it is worth setting the scene a little.

After being treated with chemotherapy for high-grade non-Hodgkin's lymphoma in 2010, I was in remission for just over two years before relapsing. This was a bit of a surprise for the doctors, as that type of high-grade lymphoma is very curable. After some investigation, and the nervous waiting that goes with the diagnosis process, it was found that the relapse was a different type of lymphoma – follicular lymphoma.

Follicular lymphoma is a low-grade disease, meaning that it is not immediately life-threatening. In fact, in many cases no treatment is needed for several years even when the disease is known to be present. In my case, however, for various reasons it did need to be treated.

The treatment I had was a slightly milder type of chemotherapy in late 2012. That pushed the disease into remission again.

The sting in the tail was that even though it's low-grade, follicular lymphoma is not ultimately curable with the normal lymphoma treatments. I was left with the knowledge that it would almost definitely come back again.

The only treatment option that seems to have a significant success rate in curing follicular lymphoma is a stem cell transplant. I was, however, told by my haematology consultants in Basingstoke that the use of stem cell transplants for follicular lymphoma was quite new and unproven. Opinion is divided on whether they should be used for low-grade lymphoma.

The lymphoma consultants in Southampton, on the other hand, evidently see it as a useful weapon in their arsenal. So I was given the option of either just harvesting my stem cells – a "rainy day" harvest – or going for the full transplant. At that stage it all felt a bit overwhelming, so I decided to go for the harvest and prepare myself mentally for having the transplant at the next relapse.

Stem Cell Harvesting

February 2013

In order to facilitate the amount of fluid and blood that would need to be given and taken during that eight- or nine-day period for the stem cell harvest, the doctor said that they would install a 'Hickman line'. That's like a PICC line, but going in through the chest, rather than the upper arm. It's a semi-permanent tube that goes through larger veins into one of the valves just above your heart. It would be left there for the duration of the procedure (and would have remained for the transplant as well if I'd decided to have that straight after).

In my case there was a two-way valve on the outside – one for in, the other for out. That's because the harvest process involves sucking the blood out, separating out stem cells, and then putting the blood back. At any one time on that day there is no more than 160 ml of blood outside the body.

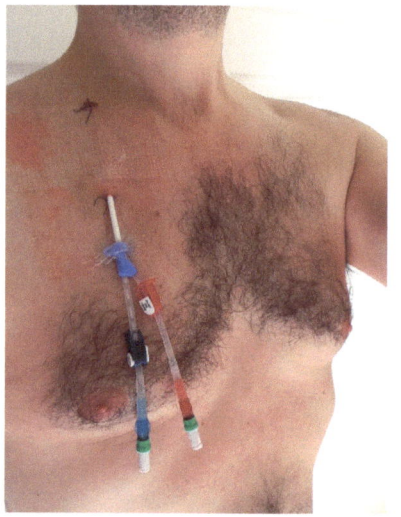

Here's a picture of my Hickman line in case you want to see exactly what I mean. It was taken just after having the line put in, so the stitches are still there. Those stitches come out after a few days, and the line stays in all by itself.

I was quite nervous about having it put in, but looking back it wasn't too bad. It was, however, another day off work, which I could have done without.

The reason it's a day off work is that even after the procedure is complete and you can go home, the advice is to avoid driving because it can be sore with the seatbelt across the collarbone just where the line is sitting.

I had to go down to Southampton Hospital (on 14th February) to have the line fitted. It's done with the aid of an x-ray, and under a local anaesthetic. So you enter an operating theatre and lie on the slab, which is then adjusted into position with the x-ray machine above it. The doctor (normally a radiologist) makes two incisions, and pushes the tube into the vein through the one next to the collarbone. The other end of the tube is then pushed under the skin to come out of the lower incision. At a couple of points the x-ray machine is used to make sure that the tube is in the right place. Sound uncomfortable? It is a bit. It's not something that I'd want to do for fun. But it was over in a couple of minutes, and the whole thing was complete fairly quickly.

I had my line in for about five weeks altogether. Often patients will have them for much longer. Every week the line needed to be flushed clean by a nurse. If I wasn't in hospital for any other reason in a particular week I had to make an arrangement for this to be done. Not a big thing (about half an hour or so), but more added hassle.

After a week or so the soreness had eased, and I hardly noticed that the tubes were there. The times that they most got in the way for me were during the night in bed when they dangled annoyingly, and in the morning when I had a shower. Having a bath wasn't allowed, as the tubes should not be submerged in water. But in order to have a shower the tubes have to be wrapped in cling film to keep them dry.

In order to get the stem cells (which are the basic cells from which all the different types of blood cells grow) out of my body they had to first be 'mobilised'. Blood cells are made in the bone marrow, and therefore that is where stem cells normally reside. However, they can come out into the blood stream, and that's where they are taken from when they harvest stem cells for a transplant. But in order to get enough stem cells they have to 'mobilise' them to come out into the blood stream in large enough volume.

To mobilise the stem cells two things are done. First a high dose of cyclophosphamide is given over the course of a day. That's one of the chemo drugs that I'd had before – the 'C' in R-CHOP and R-CVP. But in this case, they told me my hair would almost definitely fall out. After that, every day for the following week, I would have to give myself GCSF (growth factor) injections. Then I would go back to hospital and have my stem cells taken (provided that a blood test showed there were enough there). And if they didn't get enough stem cells on that day, I'd have to go back the next day (and the next, etc.), until enough cells had been harvested.

The cyclophosphamide treatment to prime the stem cells (18th February) was pretty uneventful. It took just over half a day. We were in a nice private room in Southampton Hospital with a TV. And the Hickman line worked like a dream. No messing around with needles trying to cannulise. Just connect up and start the drip!

I was back to work the next day, feeling a little tired, maybe a little sick. But nothing major.

I was told that I would almost definitely lose my hair within two to four weeks... I know it sounds stupid, but it was quite a significant thing for me. Not because I've got a particular thing about my hair, but because it's so visible. It's almost like sudden baldness is a way of saying to the world, "Hey I've got cancer and I have to have chemotherapy!" I'd been getting by at work without having to talk about my illness all the time, because when I was in the office I always looked pretty healthy. No one would have known by looking at me that I was having cancer treatment. But once I was told that my hair was going to fall out I felt I had to warn people, so that it wouldn't be a shock....

And then it didn't happen! So that created even more of a talking point! But it felt like I'd drawn attention to myself, which is not my way! Even two months later people at work were still saying, "So your hair still hasn't fallen out!"

But why was I complaining anyway? It was such a cold winter that it was good to have hair!

Anyway, the priming was on a Monday, and I was booked to start to the cell collection the following Monday (25th Feb). On the days in between I had to inject myself twice a day with GCSF, which boosts white cell growth. That honestly sounds worse than it is. It's not painful at all. The pinprick for the injection is a little tickle that sometimes aches a tiny bit afterwards! It's just a case of mind over matter to make your hand prick yourself in your stomach fat with the needle.

I warned my colleagues at work that the stem cell harvest could take a week, since I was told that can sometimes happen. So I cleared my diary and prudently prepared to be off for the week.

The reason it can take so long is that there is a certain number of cells required for a transplant. They do a blood test at the start that gives an indication whether they will be able to get enough. If not, you have to go home and have another GCSF injection and come back the next day. Then after the day's harvesting is completed they send the cells to the lab and they check to see if there are enough. If not, you have to come back the next day to do the same again.

It's a fascinating process: blood coming out of one end of the Hickman line, going into a big centrifuge (which looks a bit like one of those top-loading washing machines) where the layer containing the stem cells is removed into a bag, and then going back into the other end of the Hickman line.

In practical terms, being the one connected to the machine is fairly tedious. I was fortunate that they collected more than double the number of cells they needed in just one day. You literally sit on the bed, connected to the machine, all day – five hours. No moving around in that time, so if you need the toilet they have to bring you a bed pan – I was fortunate that I didn't need it!

One of my main issues was that if I turned or moved my head too much then the line under my skin pinched against my collarbone and reduced the flow of blood out to the machine. So I had to be fairly still and breathe evenly. That meant I couldn't really have a sleep or get too animated in conversation!

The other thing I found was, as they'd warned me, I started to suffer mild calcium deficiency. That's because the anti-coagulant, that they put in the blood as it goes through, uses up calcium. The symptoms are that you start to feel like you're vibrating or a little numb. I initially thought it was the centrifuge humming and vibrating on the floor, but I was told it was actually my body having thousands of tiny muscle spasms from depletion of calcium. The nurses are pretty relaxed about this, and they just give you some calcium tablets – it's such a common side effect that the tablets are kept in a cupboard next to the bed.

The nurses were great. Unusually, I was the only one in the room, with the constant supervision of two nurses. Normally apparently there are two or three people having stem cell collection at any one time, especially on a Monday.

We chatted about all sorts of things. One of the things they talked about was the stem cell transplant itself. They described the isolation rooms that are used, and comforted me that isolation was nowhere near as grim as it sounded.

Anyway, with the harvest done, I decided not to go straight back to work, but take a couple more days off just to rest and recover. Not that it was physically strenuous, but it had been an emotional drain.

When the "Rainy Day" Came

May 2015

After having my stem cells harvested, and I'd had the Hickman line removed, I moved onto a maintenance treatment regime, which involved having an infusion of Rituximab once every two months for two years. That treatment, I was told, increases remission from follicular lymphoma by 50% on average. So in my head I was thinking that if the first remission had been two years, then I could expect around three years until the next relapse.

But in actual fact, the next relapse came only two years later. There was a bit of a painful story around the way it was diagnosed, and that rollercoaster ride in the middle of 2015 made me more determined to have the stem cell transplant and try to get rid of the lymphoma once and for all. I won't talk about it here. If you are interested, you can read about it either on my blog or in one of my other books. Essentially, the relapse was noticed in the routine CT scan at the end of the two years of maintenance treatment, and confirmed with a biopsy.

The treatment plan that was eventually settled upon involved another different type of mild chemotherapy called Bendamustine. That would take about three to four months. The plan was to use that to get me into remission again, and then to talk about the stem cell transplant after that.

So when we pick up the transplant story again in the next chapter, I've finished my course of Bendamustine and had a PET CT scan to confirm the remission of the disease.

All-Go for the Transplant

November 2015

On Monday 16th November 2015 I went for my appointment at the Southampton Hospital Oncology department. I met with one of the consultants and the transplant co-ordinator, the same people I met back at the beginning of 2013 when my stem cells were harvested.

Just as he had done in 2013, he talked about options, which were:

1. Do three more cycles of Bendamustine and then wait for the lymphoma to come back. That would be the least intrusive, but the remission would probably only be about 12 months.
2. Autologous stem cell transplant, which is what we'd been mentally preparing for. He still said there would be a 50% chance of a total cure (greater than 10 years of remission). He made me aware of the potential complications – the chance of picking up infections, some of them potentially serious. He mentioned again that 1% of people die of infections as a direct result of the high dose chemo, but this time he acknowledged that the risk in my case would be much lower because I am young, fit and strong.
3. Allogeneic stem cell transplant. That's the same procedure except using somebody else's donated stem cells. With this one the chances of success are higher. But the risk of death is also higher, because of the risk of my body rejecting someone else's cells. And the fatality risk is significant (more than 10%).

So we confirmed that the plan we'd spoken about before was still the right plan. Autologous stem cell transplant. The allogeneic version is something he said that we could keep in reserve for "if we get in a tight spot at a later date".

The idea was that they should have had the results of the PET-CT scan (that I'd had a few weeks earlier), but they hadn't been reported yet. If those were all clear we'd be able to go ahead with the transplant. If the scan showed any lymphoma activity, then I'd be given one more round of Bendamustine before going ahead with the transplant.

As far as timing was concerned, this is where there was a bit of a surprise for me. I'd evidently started to convince myself that they would book me in for January, whilst verbally acknowledging the chance it could be sooner. So it took me a while to digest the words, "if the PET scan's ok then we should be able to get you in in a couple of weeks!"

Anticipating the question that was written all over my face, the doctor said, "you're going to ask me if we can wait until after Christmas, but I don't think we should do that." His reasoning was firstly that there will always be reasons to wait. More importantly, though, the lymphoma was coming back (albeit slowly) all the time, so it made more sense to try to consolidate my remission as quickly as possible.

But that meant that I was likely to be in hospital for Christmas, and definitely on my daughter Anna's 13th birthday (22nd December). As I called Heidi after the appointment to tell her the news, it crossed my mind that it wouldn't be the first Christmas I'd ruined (2009 being the other obvious one, but I was also recalling that I was made redundant in December 2001, again in December 2005 and again in December 2007)!

The next day, I got a call to say that the PET scan results were reported – all fine. So the wheels were set in motion to get me in for the transplant.

The kids took the news surprisingly well, partly, I think, because they knew it was coming. They were obviously disappointed about my probably absence for Christmas. Anna brought tears to my eyes. When I told her she just gave me a massive hug, smiled and said, "Dad, I don't mind that you won't be around for my birthday or Christmas Day. I'm just happy they're going to make you better."

There was lots to think about, lots to prepare (finances being one of the big ones) and lots of people to tell. In the meantime, I had to try to extricate myself from work, leaving the insanely busy project to be finished off by others. And I only had a few days to do it.

Hugs and Handshakes

An exact date was not set for the transplant until the day they wanted to admit me! I guess that's to be expected if you think about it. They have to wait for a bed to be available, and beds in the transplant ward don't become available until someone is discharged after their transplant, which is not something they can predict in advance. I didn't even know the *approximate* date until I got a letter a few days before the end of November. All I knew was that it would be "in the next couple of weeks", and that I had some tests to undergo and had to come back for another meeting with the consultant and transplant coordinator before it could go ahead.

So the 14 days between the first oncology appointment and the end of the month were really busy.

I had a bunch of tests on 19th November. I went and did some work in the office in the morning and then spent the afternoon down the road in Southampton Hospital (it's about 15 minutes' drive from where I was working) having a lung function test, a kidney function test and an echocardiogram. It took the whole afternoon, and there was quite a lot of sitting around waiting, but every single element of the tests (six appointments spread throughout the afternoon) ran exactly on time (which is remarkable!).

I did most of the Christmas shopping (good ol' Amazon) earlier than normal to save Heidi having to do it while I was in hospital. And I put the Christmas decorations up at home – again, earlier than normal, because they couldn't have done it without me.

And I arranged some financial assistance for my period of being unable to work. I approached the Chartered Accountants Benevolent Association (CABA) again, as in 2010, and they very kindly agreed to provide us with some regular money. I had to wait until I'd finished work to apply for state benefits, so I was still finishing off the application form on the day I went into hospital. And, knowing that I had quite a bit of tax due at the end of January, I had to phone HMRC[2] and explain the situation so that I could make arrangements to pay later.

There were also bits of shopping to do for things I needed for hospital, and I had to catch up on the many little odd jobs that needed to be ticked off the list if I was going to be incapacitated for a few months.

I agreed 30th November as my last day at work. I didn't know exactly when I was going into hospital, but the end of the month seemed to have some logic to it, even though it meant finishing on a Monday. It caught up on me quickly because of being so busy. And it was a little emotional, I have to admit, but lovely to feel the appreciation for my contribution to various projects and improvements over the previous four-and-a-half years.

I finished at 1pm, met Heidi at the railway station and we drove to Southampton Hospital, 15 minutes away. We had to see the consultant again to go through the plan and sign the consent form. All the test results were very good. Basically I was fit and healthy, which ironically made it the best time to do the stem cell transplant.

---

[2] Her Majesty's Revenue and Customs

Still, even in the late afternoon, they couldn't give an exact date for the transplant. All we knew was that I had to go back to Southampton to have a Hickman line fitted the next morning, and that I could be admitted any time after that. The advice was to pack and bring my suitcase just in case a bed came available.

The Stem Cell Transplant

December 2015

One of the first things that springs to my mind as I think back on my autologous stem cell transplant (bearing in mind that as I write not even two months have passed since then) is how little I remember without forcing myself. It's weird. I wonder if that's because it was such a discrete and different experience, even though it lasted for almost a month, that my brain can't match the memories with the categories of my current temporal experience. I'm glad I wrote a journal and I'm glad I took photos.

The Hickman line

On 1st December 2015 I turned up at Southampton Hospital first thing in the morning to have my Hickman line fitted. I had a Hickman line for the stem cell harvest early in 2013, but I'm sure it hurt quite a bit more this time round to have it fitted. As the radiologist was explaining that he was making a tunnel under the skin for the tubes to go through, it felt just about as uncomfortable as it sounds, even with plenty of local anaesthetic. There was a lot of pulling at the skin on my neck, and for a few minutes it felt like he was pushing hard against my throat under my skin. And after clenching my fist in pain at one point I remember thinking how soothing it was when one of the nurses noticed and started to hold and stroke my hand. Pain relieving drugs are great, but a simple human touch has its place too, and the great thing about that is that it doesn't take any training!

More than three weeks later it was quite an effort for the ward doctor to remove as well. The thing had stuck fast to the scar tissue (as it's supposed to) and took at least an hour of what felt like digging in my chest to finally pull it out. And it's left quite a scar now that it's healed up.

In between it worked really well. Whenever I needed something to be infused into me, or blood to be taken from me, there was no messing with cannulas and needles. It was simply: connect the line, set the pump and off we go (it is a little more involved than that, but you get the picture). The nurses were very strict in keeping the line ends clean at all times, disinfecting them before and after every use with a careful procedure which I can't describe (but I observed).

It made washing a bit awkward, I have to admit. I think back in 2013 I used cling film to cover the line ends while in the shower. In hospital this time I was given a 'press 'n' seal' sandwich bag and some tape to use each day. The first day was funny. I sealed the ends of the line in the bag and taped it to my shoulder – and it completely fell off as soon as water touched it when I got in the shower! Fortunately, I worked out a way of sealing the bag and taping it up that kept it secure for the other twenty-odd days. It crossed my mind to make a YouTube 'how to' video for the benefit of other Hickman line users, but I couldn't work out how to hold the camera and tape the bag up at the same time!!

Admission

While I was sat in bed after having my Hickman line fitted, feeling a little sorry for myself as the nurses attempted to stop some minor bleeding from the incisions, a nurse came around from the Bone Marrow Transplant (BMT) Ward to let me know that there would be a bed available for me that day, but not until the evening.

After a bit of discussion, Heidi and I decided to take the hour-long drive home and return later after the evening rush hour.

Saying goodbye to the kids for the second time that day was really hard. There were more tears than ever. I always feel it's my duty to be the one keeping it together, the rock, the one whose emotions do not get the better of him. So I was the only one not crying as I left the house, I think (apart from the grandparents, who were minding the kids while Heidi drove me to the hospital). The trouble is that it can make it seem like I don't care, when actually underneath my heart is aching. What I was trying to portray to them is that if I'm not afraid, then neither should they be. I knew we'd miss each other, but there would be visits and phone calls and it was only going to be three weeks or so. It would not be as a big a deal as they were feeling at that moment. And all the time I was secretly taking a big gulp, because I'd been apprehensive for the previous three months about how ill it was going to make me.

We got to Southampton Hospital again about an hour later, and I checked into Ward C6L, the BMT ward, around 8:40pm. But it was after midnight by the time I was fully booked in.

After finishing work the previous day, and the busyness of the previous two weeks, there hadn't been any real 'downtime'. It wasn't exactly planned, and at the time I think I would have preferred a couple of days to take a breath after finishing work. But in the end I have to admit that it worked out really well.

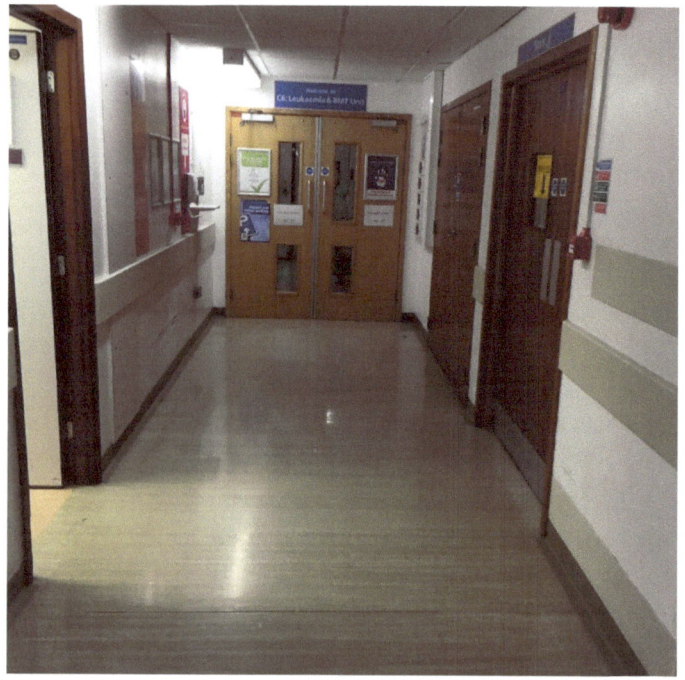

The room

When we got there we were struck by the size of the room. It was slightly smaller than I'd imagined it would be. Once I'd settled in, however, the 8 ft. by 10 ft. space, plus en-suite bathroom, was perfectly adequate. There was a TV, a fridge, a kettle, some weighing scales, some storage space and an armchair (as well as the bed of course) and free Wi-Fi! But cluttering up the place I also had the drip stand and a set of 'obs' equipment (for blood pressure, temperature, etc.). I guess that's what makes it a bit different from a hotel room!

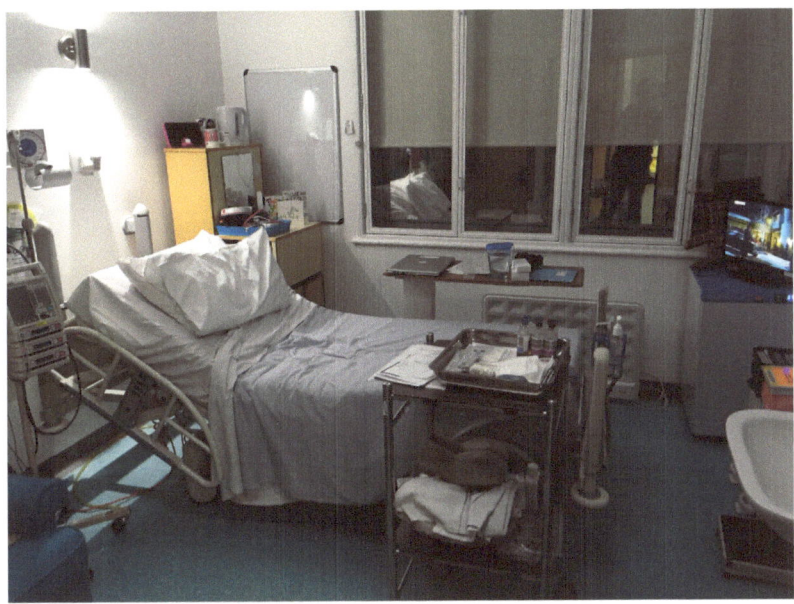

There were three whiteboards in the room, and I put two of them to use. The main one, on the wall opposite me as I lay in bed, I used for tracking things. I had to keep track of how much I was drinking (more of that later), so I would write every drink on the board. I also tracked my weight each day, and sometimes more than once a day. At the bottom of the board I ticked off whether I'd done my mouthwashes at the right times – there were two mouthwashes (one simple saline and the other, Nystatin) to do four times a day. The nurses loved all this, as it made their job easier. They would just come in and read the information off the board after checking with me that it was up to date.

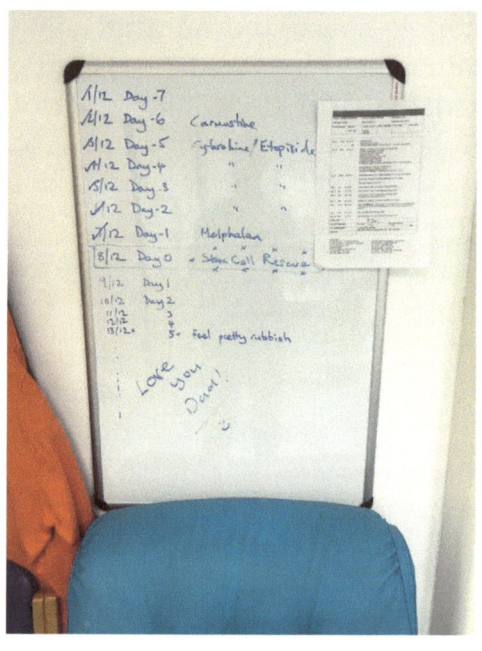

On the other board I wrote the daily treatment schedule (from the print out I'd got from one of the nurses). Six days of chemo (different drugs each day), then the stem cell transplant, then no plans except to see how I reacted and expect to feel rubbish a few days later.

The daily routine

Certain things had to be done each day.

'Obs' (that is pulse, blood oxygenation, blood pressure and temperature) would be taken six times a day, every four hours.

A typical day would begin with 6am 'obs', which could take place realistically any time between 6am and 8am, depending how busy the nurses and healthcare assistants were, and depending what else was planned for the day, treatment-wise.

Blood would be taken at the same time – they would just connect the bottles to the Hickman line. I got into the habit of asking for blood test results, at least the main figures, around midday. The nurses gave me a sheet of paper with pre-printed headings, and they got so used to me asking that some of them would just automatically come and write on my paper (which I kept stuck to my main whiteboard with Blu-Tack) without prompting. I thought it might be a hassle for them, but they were actually really happy to share the information because they liked to see me taking an interest. For my own part, I'm a numbers guy; I can't help it!

Various pills would be brought in for me by the nurses whenever they were due. I didn't keep track of what I was having or when, so I'm glad they did!

At some point each morning I'd have a visit from the catering guy, taking my order for lunch and dinner. Then a housekeeper would come and change the bedding and the towels, and a cleaner would come in and clean. And the catering staff would make sure there was tea/coffee at regular intervals, and would change my jug of specially-filtered water each morning.

So mornings weren't very good for catching up on lost sleep!

The nurses had to keep a close eye on how much fluid I was carrying. I don't fully understand the reasons for this, but it was treated with great importance. In order to do that they had to record, as I mentioned, how much fluid was going in (how much I was drinking and how much was in each bag of stuff I received via IV) and how much fluid passed out. In order to keep track of the latter I had to pee into bottles, which the nurses would regularly remove from my bathroom and weigh. My weight would also be recorded, and the nurses and doctors would check my ankles and other places, looking for signs of oedema.

Ward rounds for the doctors was mostly mid-afternoon each day, with consultants joining them twice a week.

And every evening for the first eighteen days there would be a little injection into my tummy fat. For the first eleven days the injection was some sort of anti-clotting drug, to help prevent blood clotting in my Hickman line. Once my platelet count went down below 50 that wasn't required. Then once my white cell count hit zero the daily injection was GCSF instead.

Passing the time

Heidi came to see me almost every day for a few hours. Tom and Anna (then 14 and 12) came with her on a few occasions. And Jacob (18) drove down to see me with Joe (just turned 17) once or twice too. The kids, amusingly, brought the PlayStation 3 with them when they visited, and so we had fun playing zombie games together. Heidi and I normally just chatted – together and with the ladies who normally changed my bedding and cleaned my room - and watched TV.

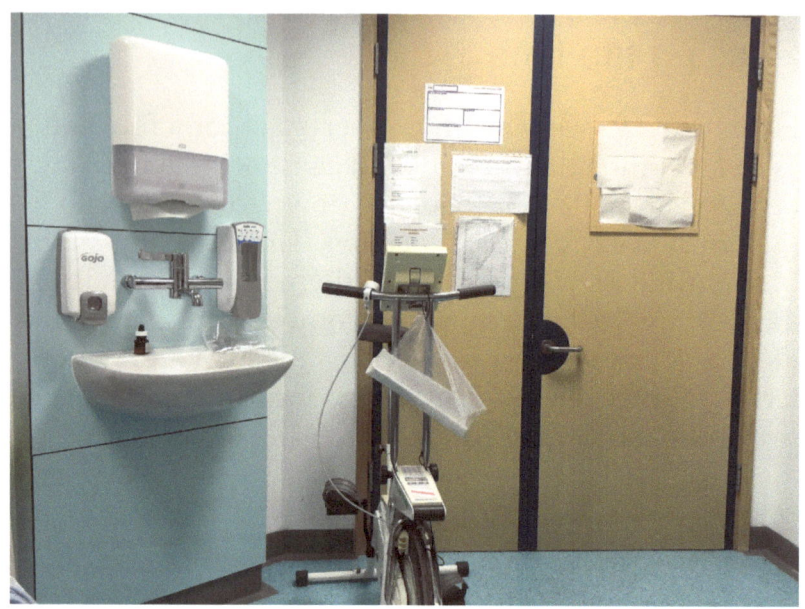

The physiotherapist came to see me on my first morning. He gave me a list of exercises to do each day. Nothing too strenuous, just things to keep the main muscles stretched and keep my heart and lungs healthy. Being confined to a small space 24 hours a day is not conducive to moving around and therefore not generally very healthy, and lying in bed a lot of the time can result in pressure sores (normally called 'bed sores'). I managed to get an exercise bike moved into my room as well.

And I did the exercises, including the bike, for about 20 minutes almost every day. Hopefully it did me some good.

I made sure every day that I made day and night distinctions. What I mean by that is that it would have been perfectly possible to spend all day and night in my pyjamas and spend the whole day in bed. But I didn't. If I wasn't connected to the IV I would shave, shower and get dressed between 6am 'obs' and breakfast. So I was always dressed and clean to start the day. And I tried to spend most of the daytime in a sitting position, either in the armchair or on the bed, unless I was specifically having a nap (which would normally be interrupted by something anyway!).

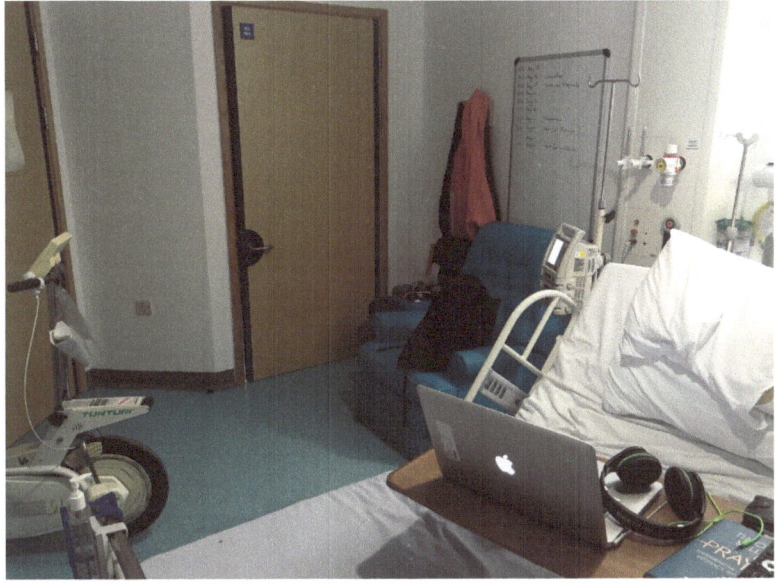

In the parts of the day when I was most alert – normally morning and early afternoon – I would read books, study the Bible and do stuff on my blog. At other times, when my brain was more tired, I would watch DVDs or occasionally watch TV. On the few days when I felt the most ill, I think I did just lay in bed most of the day, not even bothering with audio books or music. But most of the time it seemed a good thing to have a routine.

High dose chemotherapy

Treatment began as soon as I arrived. I was hooked up to IV fluids overnight and prepared for my first dose of chemotherapy, which was given around 2pm the next day.

From a treatment point of view, days are labelled in relation to the day on which the stem cells are to be infused, which is Day Zero.

Day -6 (2nd December): Carmustine. It arrived in my room and the nurse connected it up around 2pm. It took an hour to go through. I slept the whole time, for about an hour-and-a-half. Apparently that is one of the immediate effects of the drug. I was very groggy when I woke up.

Day -5 (3rd December): Cytarobine came along at 10am, taking about half an hour. Then came "hydration" (meaning a bag of saline through the drip) and two bags of Etopiside spread over two hours.

And at 9pm, as I was starting to feel nauseous for the first time really, along came the nurse with some more anti-sickness pills plus more Cytarobine. I can't remember how long the nausea lasted, but it strikes me that the reality of the situation doesn't hit until it's really real. I've had chemo before, I know how it makes you feel and what it does, and yet I was surprised when I'd had it injected and felt off colour. What did I expect?!

Day -4 (4th December): Cytarobine at 10am and 10pm, with hydration and Etopiside early afternoon.

Day -3 (5th December): Same again.

Day -2 (6th December): Same again, followed by IV fluids through the night, at a slow rate.

Day -1 (7th December): Melphalan, the last of the treatment, was infused for an hour at some stage during the day. That was then followed by another 18 hours of fluids. Melphalan is that potent.

The transplant itself

Day Zero (8th December):
The drip was on the whole night, so the combination of trying not to tangle with the line and getting up to pee about seven times meant I did not sleep well. But it wasn't as if I'd got a high pressure work day ahead. There would be plenty of time to catch up on sleep or it would catch up on me anyway!

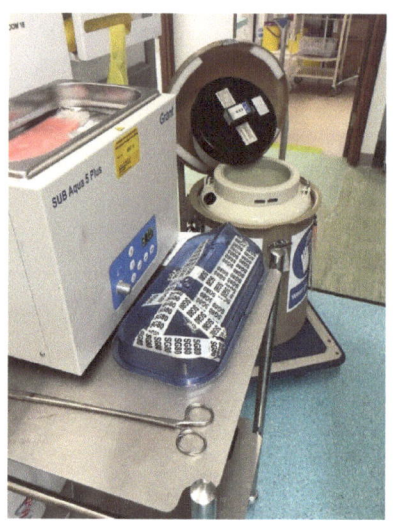

The fluids were kept going through until about 12:30pm (and so the pee bottles kept filling up all day!), and then the stem cells arrived just after lunch. There has to be at least 24 hours between the end of the chemo and the stem cell transplant.

I've heard many people say that the stem cell transplant itself is a bit of an anti-climax, because it's quite a simple, easy and quick process. But I found it all quite fascinating. The stem cells arrive in little bags of frozen pink liquid in a canister of liquid nitrogen. The nurse gets them out one at a time (using gloves) and places them in water at 38 degrees for five minutes to thaw them out. And then one by one the bags are connected to the Hickman line and infused by IV. I had six bags to get through, which I guess took about two hours.

It's quite painless. You can actually see the stem cells travelling down the line, so I was told by the nurse. They look like grains of sand. I had thought they'd be microscopic and invisible. Amazing really that they know where to go and what to do as soon as they get in the body! But then life is amazing!

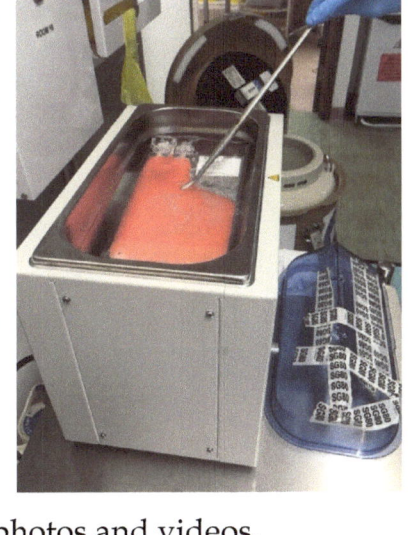

Heidi and I spent most of the two hours marvelling with the nurse and taking photos and videos.

It was a relief to be finally disconnected from the drip. I was told that I may feel sick after the Melphalan the previous day, but I wasn't too bad. I didn't feel 100%,

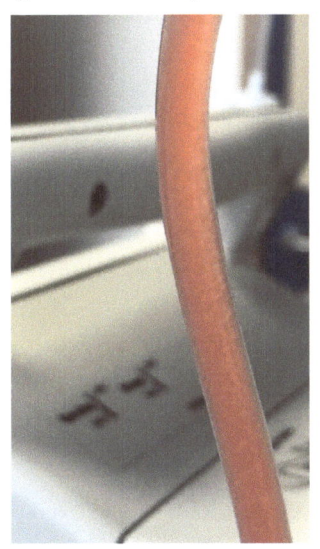

but I managed to keep smiling, hold conversation and eat food.

Because of the preservative used in the harvesting process I oozed a smell of sweetcorn for a couple of days afterwards. I couldn't smell it myself, but Heidi and Tom and Anna said that it was really strong. And because there were several patients on the ward having stem cells on the same day, the whole ward stank of sweetcorn too, so they said.

Blood counts

I said at the time that Day +1 is the anti-climax really, rather than Day Zero. No chemo, no stem cells, the drip stand pushed away, pump switched off. Just sitting around, trying to keep occupied in some way in the little room, but really just waiting for the inevitable deterioration that is due to happen within a few days.

That was really the weird part, knowing that all the treatment was done, that there was no going back, but that I was on an irreversible path towards feeling rubbish.

As I mentioned, I asked the nurses to write down the four key blood counts each day for me when the results came back:

- Hb (Haemoglobin) – indication of red blood cells
- Plt (Platelets) – cells to aid clotting
- WCC (White Cell Count) – broad immune system indicator
- Neut (Neutrophils) – particular type of white anti-infection cells

On Day +1, for instance, all my levels were still within a normal range, except for platelets, even though they were all already trending downwards. My WCC was 4.5 (against a 'normal' range of 4-11). Neutrophils were 4.3 (against a 'normal' range of 2.0-7.5).

Because my disease is lymphoma, it affects the white cells. So the aim of the high dose chemo is to reduce the WCC and 'neut' counts to zero – yes, absolutely nothing. Other blood cells do suffer as well – hence the risk of bleeding/bruising (low platelets) and the exhaustion (anaemia – low red cells) – but not as much. And then the new stem cells will busily be engrafting and generating new cells, so that within a few days of reaching zero the counts will be picking up again.

While the WCC and 'neut' counts are zero, picking up infections is expected, and it's really just a question of how bad and how many. That's why patients are isolated with strict hygiene control.

My neutrophils hit zero on Day +5, and white cells hit zero on Day +6. White cells started to flicker into life again (up to 0.1) on Day +8, with neutrophils doing the same on Day +10. I know that the GCSF growth factor injections played a part in the white cell recovery, but I was really surprised how quickly the WCC and 'neut' counts recovered. By Day +10, they were both at the lower end of the normal range (5.5 and 3.7, respectively). I was expecting them to creep up gradually and to be still below normal when I left hospital.

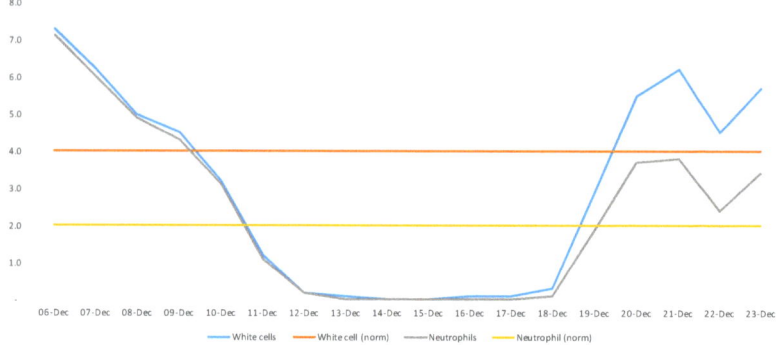

Andy Burrows - WCC and 'neut' during autologous stem cell transplant

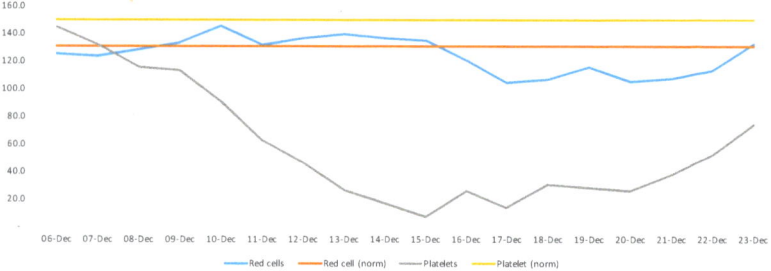

Andy Burrows - platelets and Hg during autologous stem cell transplant

Side effects

By Day +3 (11th December) I was definitely starting to feel the strain on my body. Tummy ache and going to the toilet were the main problems initially. I thought at the time it might have been the first sign of infection, and they took samples (poor things) to check. But the doctor told me that it was actually more likely to have been the chemo drugs themselves playing havoc with my digestive system.

Fatigue was also catching up, probably partly because the aches and pains were preventing me from sleeping as much as I needed to.

Day +3 was also when I started to go off my food. This is something they predict, and everybody I've read about goes through a period when they simply don't want to eat. For me, the altered sense of smell and taste made it difficult to enjoy anything really – even the simple cheese and ham sandwich I ordered for lunch. I couldn't even face a simple cup of coffee, and preferred to stick to water.

On Day +4 (12th December) I woke with a headache, and my tummy felt bad all day. My mouth felt sore, but strangely didn't have any ulcers. And I was generally just washed out. I wasn't eating at all, because I literally could not face any food. The thought of it even made me feel sick.

Some of the nurses and doctors were more concerned than others about me not eating, and they encouraged me to at least have nutritional milkshakes, which I was fortunately able to stomach. They reckoned they'd have to give me an NG (nasogastric) tube to get food directly into my stomach if I didn't eat enough. Having had an NG tube before (during my 2010 hospital stay) I was therefore motivated to try and eat, or at least have milkshakes, in order to avoid that! However, a few of the doctors, and the consultants in particular, said that they weren't terribly worried and didn't want me to stress about it, especially since the levels of nutrients in my blood (e.g. potassium, calcium, iron, etc.) remained normal the whole time.

And when people said to me that at this stage all I would feel like doing is lying around doing nothing, they were not far from the truth. That's pretty much exactly what I did most of the time for several days.

By Day +6 (14th December) things were still getting worse. I was at my most vulnerable too, so I was aware that things could get even worse quite quickly.

When I got up for the toilet in the night I came over with a cold sweat and almost passed out, and I just lay in bed most of the day. Most of the time I couldn't even muster the enthusiasm to put the TV on or listen to music. Heidi was very patient when she visited, but it must have been very boring for her!

Thankfully I perked up enough to watch a film and chat on FaceTime on separate occasions with Heidi, Tom and Anna in the evening. But it left me quite drained.

By Day +7 (15th December) I had almost constant discomfort, bordering on pain, in my gut. It felt like bad heartburn or indigestion. Apparently this is expected, and is due to the Melphalan, the most potent of the chemo drugs I've had. The consultant's comment, when he did his rounds, was that, "yes we do try to make it as much of an ordeal as possible for you!" But he reassured me nonetheless that everything I was experiencing was exactly what they expected, and in a matter of a week or so I would start to feel better, even if I got a bit of a temperature and had to have IV antibiotics along the way.

And at 10pm obs, just as he'd predicted, my temperature was up to 37.7C. That meant there were a bunch of samples to be done to isolate where the infection was, and in the meantime IV antibiotics three times a day for the following seven days.

The consultant asked how I was holding up mentally. Apparently around that point it's common for people to start questioning whether they will ever feel better, or whether they'll be stuck in isolation feeling rubbish for a long time. So he guaranteed that it would only be a few more days before I started feeling a bit better, and that I would make a full recovery.

I can't say that that had crossed my mind. I'm a trusting sort, and as far as I could analyse (even at the time) I was experiencing everything they told me to expect, perhaps even towards the better end of scale. But it did *feel* like such a long time at the time. I would think silly things like how I would love to feel the outside air on my face, enjoy a pizza, or any food for that matter, not have to pee into bottles(!), be at home with the Christmas decorations and my comfy bed, not to mention to be with Heidi and the kids milling around in the normal busyness of everyday life. There were so many things I missed, being cooped up in that room. Only a little bit longer, just a little longer.

Coming into Day +8 (16th December) I didn't sleep well. The pain in my gut and my headache started to come back half way through the night, once the Codeine and Paracetamol had worn off. It was probably the most painful night I had, and I felt quite sorry for myself in the morning.

At 6am, with the routine blood tests and 'obs', I was given the next dose of antibiotics. And it was then that the nurse also had the idea of giving me soluble Paracetamol instead of pills. That actually worked very well, and really helped to dampen the pain in my gut as well as dull the headache. It at least allowed me to feel human enough to go and have a shower and get dressed for the day.

And as the day progressed I felt much better (maintained by soluble Paracetamol). I certainly had a smile on my face and was able to sit chatting with Heidi when she came for the afternoon and evening.

I had a chest x-ray in the morning – one of those tests to isolate where the infection is/was. It was a treat to see the outside of my room, as I was pushed in a wheelchair through the busy hospital corridors to the x-ray theatre. Of course, I was wearing a mask to prevent breathing in germs, which made me look a little strange.

It was also adjudged that I had not been peeing enough! In other words, I hadn't drunk enough in the previous day, when it was important to keep things washing through my system. I tried hard, but swallowing was difficult, and I genuinely thought I'd drunk enough. Perhaps I actually sweated more than I thought when I had a temperature? Or maybe I should have just drunk more when they told me to. Anyway, the upshot was that I was connected to the drip again for constant fluid intake, and was on it overnight.

On Day +9 (17th December) I spent the morning feeling tired and lounging around doing nothing.

I'd made up my mind I was going to try to eat. The smell of the food no longer put me off, and I thought it was worth a try. However, after a few bites of toast I couldn't manage any more because my throat was so sore. It was a real painful effort swallowing. I managed one mouthful of pizza at lunchtime, and a small amount of chicken casserole and mashed potato at dinner. Thankfully the jelly and yoghurt was regaining its taste!

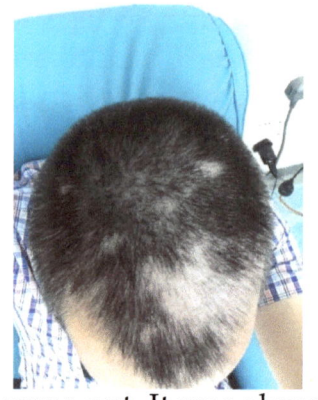 My hair started to come out on Day +9 as well, but only in the sense that I could pull out clumps of hair from my head. Heidi found it a bit gross and so I didn't do it around her, but when I was on my own it was sometimes fun to pinch a bunch (it was only about 1cm long anyway!) and pull, and see how many hairs came out. It was always a good few!

On Day +10 (18th December) I still felt bad. My sore throat got worse during the night, so I was prescribed some Oramorph, which only just about took the edge off the pain. By the morning, with not much sleep behind me, I also had a splitting headache. I was not looking forward to a day of not being able to eat or drink much because of my throat, and I even suggested first thing in the morning that they set up the IV fluids for the day because I didn't think I'd be able to drink enough.

Fortunately, they prescribed Difflam mouthwash and that really helped to numb the pain at the back of my throat. I still didn't feel like eating, but it made the day less painful. And I was able to drink sufficient to avoid IV fluids.

Day +12 (20th December) was when I started to feel a little bit better.

I managed to do my exercises and I ate a little. I was still very tired, but felt generally more positive. And since my hair, by that stage, was really patchy, one of the nurses offered to get the clippers and shave the rest off. So Day +12 was also the day on which I went completely bald.

Waiting to go home

They never found the source of the temperature that I had on Day +7, and after that one set of 'obs' I showed no other signs of infection. So with my blood counts rapidly improving, and starting to feel a little better in myself, my mind turned even more impatiently to going home.

If it weren't for the time of year, I think I would have cared less about how long my stay was exactly. However, everything was heading towards Christmas. Everything in the outside world, that is. In my sterile little room, in my bubble, I felt cut off from any festivities. I saw the Christmas party photos on Facebook and felt left out. And I couldn't stand the thought of being in that unfestive bubble while the rest of the family were at home opening presents and having Christmas dinner on the 25th.

As it was, I had to join in Anna's 13th birthday morning celebrations via FaceTime on 22nd. And Heidi brought her and Tom to see me later on in the day, which was lovely, but not the same as being at home.

So from around Day +12 onwards the big question in my mind was, "will I be home in time for Christmas?" The consultant and the nurse specialist were pretty sure that I would. But I was then grasping for information on when exactly, what the criteria were, etc. My blood counts seemed to be ok, I was feeling ok, and eating ok, so why couldn't I go home? I was a little disappointed when I was told by one junior doctor that I had to finish the seven-day course of antibiotics before I could go home, as well as avoiding any other infections, which meant that it would be at least the 23rd.

All in all, my period of feeling really rough lasted eight or nine days starting from Day +3 or +4, and I went home at about 7:45pm on 23rd December (Day +15). I was in Southampton Hospital for 23 days altogether, which I'm told is the average stay for an autologous stem cell transplant. Everything went according to plan, and the doctors were very pleased with the way things went. For me and the family, we were just pleased I was home for Christmas!

Being cared for

During the whole hospital stay we were amazed at people's generosity. For instance, I mentioned Heidi's travel and parking costs one day in my daily blog journal, and a couple of people just sent us money to cover it.

One of the biggest helps for Heidi was our church arranging evening meals every day for her and the kids, so that she didn't have to worry about that while thinking about everything else. One of the ladies arranged a rota so that over the course of the month eight or ten people took turns to prepare and deliver a meal for the family almost every day of the week.

There were also spontaneous gifts via PayPal, cash and bank transfer from several family members and friends. I sat thinking at one stage how I didn't deserve such gifts, but also knowing that we would have struggled severely to get by without them (even with the help of CABA).

So we were extremely grateful to all those who found it in their hearts to help us financially and practically, but also to those who prayed and listened and had the time and sensitivity to just 'be there'.

It also really lifted my spirits to have people say that they were actually interested in hearing my daily thoughts. For the stem cell transplant I posted my daily journal on my blog as part of the *Cancer and Me* series. And I set it up to auto-update my status on Facebook and Twitter when I posted a new entry. And it became more interactive than I had anticipated. I had many lovely messages of encouragement, from friends, from family, from friends I haven't spoken to for years, and from friends of friends and family! We were really blessed. I was touched, and more than a little bit surprised, that so many people cared so much as to be interested in hearing from me daily.

I don't think I can say 'thank you' enough to all those who followed, cared, helped where possible, prayed, encouraged, and cheered us on during my stay in hospital. As I was saying my goodbyes in the office at the end of November 2015 I was preparing myself mentally for quite a lonely period, with me in isolation, and with Heidi and the kids struggling on without me at home. But it was not like that at all, and we were so blessed through so many different people from all over the place (and indeed all over the world via the internet).

May God bless them all, and I hope that we have chance to pay back and pay forward some of the blessings that we've received in the future.

One of the things that struck me was that often people commented on the positivity in my journal entries. But I hadn't realised I was being positive! I thought I was just "telling it how it is"! The funny thing was that simply being told that I sounded positive made me *feel* more positive! There's a lesson in that somewhere – simple words of encouragement and appreciation have a big impact.

The other lesson is that sharing our experiences and feelings in intense hard times was worthwhile. I did it to help others who come after me, so that they would know the kind of thing to expect if they have to go through a stem cell transplant. What I hadn't expected was how richly and immediately that investment would return to me in words of encouragement and love. I'd recommend other cancer sufferers consider blogging if they feel they can, or at least don't shy away from sharing what you're going through with your friends on Facebook or Instagram or whatever.

The only other thing that remains to mention about the stay in hospital for the stem cell transplant is that the staff were great.

Obviously I am primarily referring to the nursing staff, some of whom I got to know better than others. From the two hospital stays in my adult life I think that nurses in general are amazing. They have some really unpleasant jobs to do, and they see their patients at their worst, or at least at their most vulnerable. All of the nurses I met were utterly professional in doing their work carefully (e.g. the number of times they have to remember to put on and take off gloves, wash hands, change aprons, disinfect lumens, flush lines; e.g. having patience with temperamental drip pumps, blood pressure cuffs, etc.). And they all really care. Some of the nurses, even some of the young trainee nurses, would come in and chat and make sure I was ok, and would even check on Heidi if she was visiting.

But it's not just nurses. I was struck by the team effort it takes to run a ward like the BMT ward. The healthcare assistants, the housekeepers, the cleaners, the caterers, and not forgetting the doctors. And it's not as if they each have their jobs and they stick to them, and it all works like clockwork. It's a lot more dynamic than that thankfully. Even the catering manager, the housekeepers and the cleaners, amongst others, would stop for a chat with us, listen and give us words of encouragement. All of them were used to seeing people come in, have their chemo, receive their stem cells, go off their food, turn very poorly and incommunicative, and leave with no hair. And to emphasise the point, I was pleased to observe the odd student doctor work shadowing with the cleaners and housekeepers.

I don't think it's possible to underestimate the positive impact and importance of the caring ethos that permeates through every role in the department, and the team effort that is required.

And therefore, I will always be extremely grateful for our National Health Service. I was so fortunate to be ill in the UK where everything I need is readily available to me. Politicians of all colours often speak as if the NHS is fundamentally broken and doesn't work. In my opinion that's rubbish. No organisation, especially one of that size, is free of problems that need to be resolved. But let's at least acknowledge how great it is to have what we've got, and try not to destroy it while we're 'fixing' it!

Last day in hospital

On my penultimate day in Southampton Hospital, Prof Johnson, the blood cancer specialist consultant, came round early in the afternoon.

As well as saying that he was happy for me to go home the next day, he gave me several bits of advice. For one thing apparently it's not unusual for transplant patients being discharged in the winter months to go home and get a chest infection straight away, and in which case he urged me not to suffer in silence, however much I wanted to avoid going back into hospital. So he also said I should "have a quiet Christmas - act like you're about 20 years older!"

The other thing he predicted was that being at home would make me feel "wiped out" for a while. He couldn't explain why, but even though I was feeling fine in my little room in hospital he said everyone going home says the same. There is just something about being in normal everyday surroundings (I have a feeling there's also something to do with having had quite strong chemotherapy!). He said some people get depressed about it, but he encouraged me not to, because it's absolutely normal and after a few months I will feel much better.

Anyway, after, ironically, my best night's sleep of the whole stay, I got up on 23rd December and packed my suitcase. And then I sat and waited like an excited child sitting on his suitcase waiting to go on holiday!

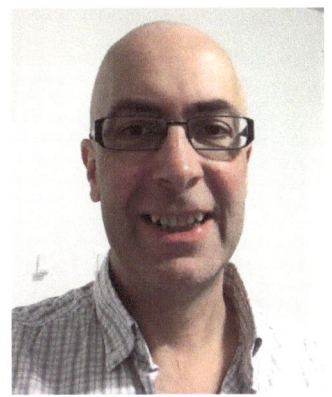

One of the transplant co-ordinators came round in the morning to go through things I needed to know about looking after myself at home. It came down to staying away from crowded places and people with illnesses, and sticking to a special diet for about six weeks. I was to have a follow up appointment on 11th January in Southampton, but for any other problems I needed to contact Basingstoke Hospital straight away. She also emphasised how tired I would feel for the following few months.

Before I was able to go home a couple of other bits needed to be ticked off the checklist. Pharmacy had to get a bunch of pills up to me to take home (the TTOs). But the main thing was that I needed to be given a prophylactic (preventative) drug for a particular type of pneumonia. That is given via a nebuliser, but it has to be done in a special room with air filtration. So it's by appointment, and my appointment was at 4pm. But they were running very late so it was more like 7pm! And by the time we got away it was around 7:30pm. In the meantime, it was just tedious waiting!

Being Home Again

My first week back at home after my stem cell transplant was tougher than we all expected (in spite of being told that it would be difficult).

For a start, on the very night I came out of hospital Heidi came down with a bug and was violently sick during the night. I was torn between wanting to get up and help her and knowing that I needed to keep clear of infectious people for my own safety. Fortunately, she wasn't sick again, but developed cold/virus symptoms which lasted a few days.

So Christmas Eve was hard work, with bits of present-wrapping left to do, as well as staying up late and carting sacks of presents up and down stairs to prepare for the morning's excitement.

Christmas Day was lovely. The kids had all bought me really fantastic presents, which made me feel really special. And Heidi's mum and dad came over and cooked Christmas dinner for us, which made it a lot less strenuous than it could have been.

My only frustration was that, because of my damaged taste buds, I could not manage to eat my normal huge portion and I couldn't taste anything, even when I covered everything in cranberry sauce!

And my limitations did get me down. The comment was made that I was chirpier in hospital, and I admit it was true. When there were things I had to do, like replacing the TV stand that broke, or helping to set up some of the kids' presents, I couldn't seem to hide how physically difficult I was finding it. It just made me come across as a bit of a grumpy old man. I tried to explain that it was easier in hospital to be chirpy for two or three hours when Heidi and the kids were visiting, and even then I would be sat in bed while chatting with them. And then when they'd gone I could immediately put my head down and have a kip without getting out of bed! That's entirely different to having to get around the house and keep up a smile for 16 hours at a time.

Two things mainly got me down. The biggest thing was my lack of taste. Everything tasted horrible. The only things that were vaguely palatable were very sweet things like trifle or ice cream (or cranberry sauce). I couldn't even stomach chocolates or cake. So I didn't tend to eat very much, and lost more weight. That was not a disaster, as I'd only lost about 6-7kg in hospital and I was still a bit overweight, but it did make me realise how much I enjoy eating food!

The other thing was my lack of energy. I knew that they warned me of this, and it was probably worse because of not eating properly. But almost every time I stood up or walked about the house I got light-headed and dizzy. Things that would normally be easy for me were really hard work. Even when I gave up and went to bed, I'd go out like a light for two whole hours, and still didn't feel any better afterwards!

It hit me that everything I'd been warned of was likely to be true. This was going to be a long recovery process.

The Long Road of Recovery

About ten days after coming home my sense of taste started to rapidly improve, to the extent that I was able to eat normally. I still had the annoying smell – a bit like dirty dishwater - lingering in my nose at least half the time. But at least food wasn't quite as bland and I could actually eat it without feeling sick.

Consequently, the light-headedness became less of an issue and I started to feel a little stronger.

About a week after that, I started to get out and about occasionally too, giving lifts to the kids in the car. And a couple of times I felt up to walking the dogs with Heidi.

The problem is that recovery doesn't progress consistently and it's slow. So the first time I went out and walked the dogs I ended up being really tired for the next few days.

It was hard explaining to the kids that it would be a slow recovery. One of the younger ones asked me in the early stages at home (during a game of Cluedo), "Dad, when are you going to get your spark back?" Personally, I never knew I had a spark in the first place! But practically speaking, I guess I knew what they meant – things like needing help taking the outdoor Christmas lights down, having to leave Heidi to take the indoor Christmas decorations down, needing someone else to do some small DIY jobs, all because I hadn't got the strength or energy.

One of my first targets was to get to the point where I could stop being careful who I saw and where I went because of the risk of infection. I thought that would be around the beginning of February. But I saw the consultant in Southampton on 11th January, and he said that my blood counts were so good and trending in the right direction that he was completely relaxed. He told me I could do whatever I felt up to, but just not to get close to people who were clearly ill. Diet-wise, I could also stop boiling the drinking water and go back to normal (the only precaution was to avoid pate and soft cheeses for another couple of months).

So I went to church on Sunday 17th January, which was the first time since November the previous year.

On the other hand, my target of building up my levels of exercise took longer to progress towards. I walked the dogs a bit more, but avoided the exercise bike and more strenuous things like sit-ups and press-ups for a long time.

I also succumbed to a mild cold (the sniffy and sneezy kind of cold) a couple of times and that really knocked the energy out of me.

So two steps forward, one-and-a-half steps back.

The consultant did say that recovery doesn't go in a straight line. He said some days would be better than others. That is true. And it means you can't perceive any improvement if you compare day to day, or even week to week, progress.

I was discharged from the care of the specialist lymphoma team in Southampton to the care of my old familiar team of haematologists in Basingstoke. And I was prescribed two kinds of pills to take for six months:

- Aciclovir – to prevent shingles. Apparently, the chemo can make patients very susceptible to shingles.
- Co-Trimoxazole (Septrin) – this is to prevent a particularly nasty type of chest infection which can be fatal. The doctor said that he'd never known anyone get that infection if they've taken the pills for the whole 6 months, but it is a danger if I don't. So I resolved to take the pills!

When I saw one of my haematology doctors on 27th January I was told I was doing very well, and that I ought to have a break from hospital. So he didn't want to see me again for three months. The last time I'd had three months between appointments was in 2012!

As I put the finishing touches to my first two books at the end of February 2016, I was just starting to get my hair back, although I was still shaving it off once a week so that it would grow back evenly. There were other things, side effects that, though not of any concern, were just odd. Things like dry skin on my hands and face – to the extent that my finger prints disappeared and I couldn't use TouchID on my iPhone! Things like the ridges that appeared on my fingernails.

But the main thing was tiredness, or energy levels to be more precise. I gradually struggled less to get out of bed in the morning, and I could get through a morning of dog walking and other chores as I would normally. But around lunchtime I would "hit the wall", and my batteries would need recharging with an afternoon nap. There were busy days when I managed to force myself to get through a whole day without a rest, but I ended up flaked out by the end of them, and it was a while before I could do it several days in a row.

So there was a weird few months, similar to the latter part of 2010, when there were no treatment and no hospital trips, no feeling ill. Just waiting - waiting to recover to an extent where work is viable.

How could I gauge that? If I were in a permanent job, and had taken time off sick, I might have discussed a way of going back part time to ease myself in. But as a self-employed consultant or interim manager, work would most likely to be full time or not at all, and I had to be able to offer myself confidently for a new assignment as soon as I was ready. It was just impossible to predict when that would be.

So I kept myself occupied with writing[3] and monitoring my energy levels, and aimed to make a proper self-assessment of my capabilities late in April. After that I could see my treatment recovery transitioning seamlessly into the other standard trial in my life – unemployment.

---

[3] I self-published *Cancer and Me*, in March 2016, and *Facing Cancer with Faith* the month after that. Find out more at www.andyburrows.me.

Rounding Off

As it happened, the unemployment didn't happen. I suddenly, quite unexpectedly, had a day early in May 2016 where I didn't get tired and got through a day of normal activities. And by the end of the month, not only was I feeling ready to go back to work, but I had the offer of a full time six-month contract back at the place I'd worked before my transplant.

It turns out that the doctors were pretty much exactly right. It took six months to be well enough to be back at work full time. And since then I haven't looked back. It's now September 2016. And there have been many times when I've been walking around the office and I marvel that I feel normal, as if that six months never happened. Many days I find myself looking back, thinking that I feel better than I have done for ages – since before my relapse was diagnosed nearly 18 months ago.

Obviously I know that some people take longer to feel normal after a stem cell transplant. So if you're approaching a stem cell transplant as you read this, I can't promise your experience will be exactly like mine. However, you should be encouraged by my experience that normal life is possible. Who knows? I may even be free of lymphoma forever. But even if not, I am enjoying the current health and strength that the stem cell transplant has given me.

I'm now being told that I should focus on getting my fitness and "heart health" up. Chemo can have a detrimental effect on your heart, even though being fairly young I may not feel it. But it will help me in the long run to exercise and stay fit.

Final words of advice?

Firstly, don't be afraid. It seems like a very intense treatment, and physically gruelling. And it is. But you will have doctors and nurses there with you every step of the way, and they will tell you each step as you need to face it, and they know what they're doing and what to expect. They know how to relieve whatever pain and discomfort you may feel. And they'll do everything they can to make it as comfortable as possible.

Secondly, take only one step at a time. With the process mapped out, as it is in the hospital information you will have received, and as it is in this book, you know what to expect almost day by day. But you only know from words on a page, so I know you will still be anxious for the experience itself. But you only need to focus on each step as it comes. The next appointment, the admission, today's chemo, and so on. People sometimes say to me, "How did you cope?" And I just say, "by putting one foot in front of the other and keeping moving." Just focus on doing what you need to do today, and leave the future to take care of itself.

Thirdly, don't be afraid to share how you are feeling with anyone around you during the process. If you feel sick, if you have a headache or a sore throat, if you feel faint, if you don't feel like eating or sleeping or talking, if you feel emotional – tell a nurse, or a doctor, or the cleaner or catering manager or one of your visitors. You don't have to act tough. People want to help, and they want to cheer you on. So let your family and friends know how you're doing. Their words of encouragement will mean more to you than you understand right now.

Finally, don't be discouraged if your recovery feels slow afterwards. In my experience the progress made day by day is almost imperceptible. But over time you will notice the small things. First you recover your sense of taste and appetite. Then you may be able to go for walks and do normal activities in the morning. For weeks on end you will find you need to go back to bed during the day. After a while those naps will feel more like just resting in bed, without falling asleep. That doesn't mean you didn't need to rest. It just means your body needed to pause rather than shut down and restart.

I found after a while it was a bit like having a battery with a short life. I could get up early, do normal activities, but then I'd grind to a halt and need to recharge. Eventually, I unexpectedly came to a day when the battery lasted all day. It didn't mean the next day would be the same. But I knew on that day that I was nearly there.

So don't rush yourself. Don't be impatient. Remember everything you've been through. Your body was slammed with a lethal dose of poisonous drugs that would have killed you if it hadn't been for the medical professionals and the "stem cell rescue" on Day Zero. It will take time. Allow yourself that time to recover fully before stepping back into frenetic normal activity.

Blessing

So it only remains for me to wish you every blessing as you face this significant part of your battle with your disease.

If you contact me via my website (andyburrows.me) I will pray for you personally. But I pray now for whoever reads this book while looking forward to your own transplant, that you would have a successful transplant with no complications. I pray that you will be free from anxiety, and that you would know "the peace of God that transcends all understanding". Ultimately I pray that your experience will lead you to a big picture perspective on life that is only found in Jesus Christ[4].

---

[4] And if you want to find out more about that perspective through my own experience, you can read more in my book, *Facing Cancer with Faith*.

About the Author

Andy Burrows lives in Basingstoke in England. He is married to Heidi, and has four children – Jacob, Joe, Tom and Anna. After qualifying as an accountant, he moved to be a Finance Manager in a big bank, and since then has held senior Finance roles in businesses as diverse as software, utilities and financial services. Nowadays he acts as a consultant and interim manager, 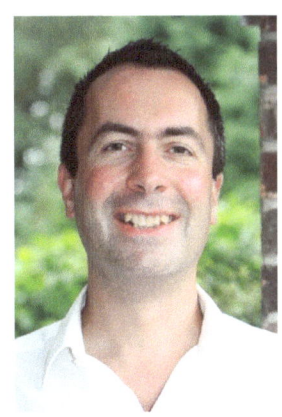 helping businesses with Finance projects, and runs a website for business Finance people – www.superchargedfinance.com.

He is also a three-time cancer survivor, author and blogger. You can find out more about Andy at www.andyburrows.me.

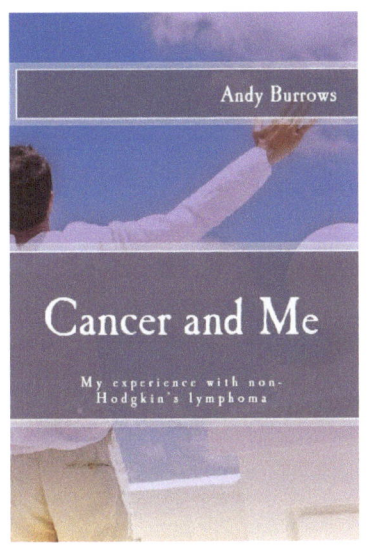

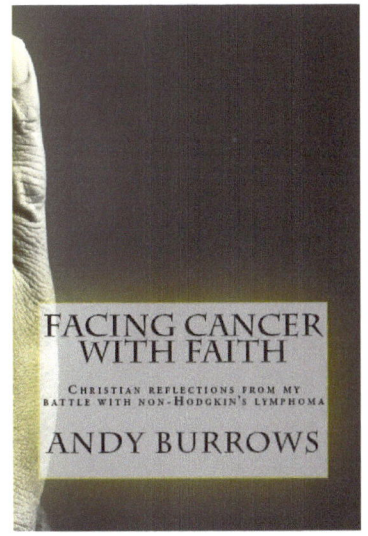